Take Control of Your CHOLESTEROL

The most comprehensive ways of taking charge of your cholesterol through low-oxalates foods. (Maintain the good[HDL] and eliminate the bad[LDL])

John C. Neely

Table of contents

Introduction

Struggling with a high level of Cholesterol? Struggle no more, here is the answer.

Cholesterol can be regarded as an important component of our bodies. But however, a high level of cholesterol can put you at a very significant risk of various types of health issues. Diseases such as stroke, heart disease etc are diseases associated with a high level of cholesterol.

When cholesterol is too much in the body, it will eventually contribute to the development of heart disease which stands as a major cause of death globally. However, many people globally are struggling with high levels of cholesterol and are also finding means to reduce their cholesterol level while eating well and maintaining a balanced diet.

As a person, it is important for you to be adequately familiar with the detriment of high cholesterol levels and the danger they cause.

One of the best ways of controlling your cholesterol levels is to develop a disciplinary mindset on the intake of nutritious and well-balanced diets. You need foods that are low in cholesterol.

Are you interested in lowering your high cholesterol levels while keeping to a healthy diet? In this book you will learn about foods to take and foods you should avoid.

This book is a very powerful book that provides the readers with the best and finest foods list that you can consume to naturally lower your cholesterol levels while maintaining a balanced diet.

If your health is your topmost priority, then you will have to get this book now and discover how to overcome high cholesterol levels through natural foods without breaking the bank.

Chapter one

What is cholesterol?

Cholesterol is a substance that helps your body in various ways. It's a design block of your cell films. Furthermore, it helps with the creation of chemicals, bile, and vitamin D — all of which require cholesterol. Be that as it may, having a lot of it in your blood can make you bound to get coronary illness. Cholesterol is a sort of lipid that does a ton of significant things in your body.

Lipids are substances that stay together in your blood since they don't separate in water. In light of everything; they make an excursion through your blood to show up at different bits of your body that need them. Your liver produces adequate cholesterol to meet your body's prerequisites. Be that as it may, the food varieties you eat likewise give you more cholesterol.

There is a way for your body to dispose of the overabundance of cholesterol. In any case, there are times when that framework breaks down or becomes overburdened. Therefore, you could have more cholesterol in your blood. What's more, that is the point at which you could run into issues. Cholesterol isn't terrible all alone. You should live. Notwithstanding, elevated cholesterol levels can be destructive. That is the explanation it's basic to learn about cholesterol, including its abilities and types. Understanding the reason why you want cholesterol — however not a lot of it — might benefit from some intervention by this information. It can moreover help you with understanding what your cholesterol numbers mean and how to take action to cut down them if fundamental.

What is the ability of cholesterol? Your body involves cholesterol for the vast majority of significant things. These include: helping the development of defensive layers on your cell films. What can enter or leave your cell is constrained by these layers. helping your liver in creating bile, which is essential for processing. Supporting your body's formation of explicit synthetics (counting sex synthetic substances) and vitamin D. Accepting cholesterol is key, why do I have to worry about the sum I have? It's critical to have sufficient cholesterol to address your issues. An elevated cholesterol level can have adverse consequences.

Coronary corridor sickness is bound to influence individuals who have dyslipidemia or elevated cholesterol (hyperlipidemia). All of the cholesterol your body needs to work is made by your body. In all honesty, your liver makes up around 80% of all the cholesterol in your body. The rest (which your body doesn't need) comes from your food. Customarily, your body can filter through the cholesterol it shouldn't even worry about. In any case, your body's ability to keep a sound cholesterol level can be influenced by different elements. For example, familial hypercholesterolemia and other hereditary circumstances assume a part. These circumstances frustrate your body's capacity to wipe out overabundance of cholesterol. Accordingly, after some time, it develops in your circulation system.

Your eating routine is likewise significant. Cholesterol levels can rise when you devour food sources high in soaked fat or trans fat. For you to be on the saver side, find absorbed fat things that come from animals, like meat, milk, cheddar, and spread. Trans fat is tracked down in a ton of cheap food and handled food sources. Accordingly, trying not to have an excessive amount of cholesterol in your body can be made simpler by focusing on what your eating regimen means for your cholesterol levels.

Where is cholesterol found in my body? Cholesterol particles are available in each cell in your body. Nonetheless, you are likely most acquainted with it as a blood-borne microbe. Cholesterol has a corrective substance that holds it back from traveling solo through your blood. It must be linked to additional molecules.

As a result, it collaborates with proteins and a different kind of lipid known as triglycerides. A lipoprotein is created when these molecules join together to form a particle.

How do lipoproteins work?

A lipoprotein is a protein and lipid combination that can move through your blood. Lipoproteins are like tiny boats that go from one place to another. Each town receives food and supplies from a few boats. The trash is carried away by other boats.

Lipoproteins are proteins in your body that carry cholesterol to your tissues. This cholesterol is significant for your body to work. However, too much of it is harmful. That is the reason you want different lipoproteins that get the additional cholesterol and divert it.

These lipoproteins might be known by their nicknames. LDL cholesterol and HDL cholesterol are typically their names. The two primary types of cholesterol are as follows: However, there are different sorts, as well. Therefore, let's take a closer look at the various kinds of cholesterol and the functions they perform in your body.

What are the various sorts of cholesterol?

There are many different kinds of cholesterol in your body. They will be listed in the results of your lipid panel. Realizing what each type means can assist you with discussing your cholesterol with your medical services supplier.

What is LDL cholesterol?

Low-density lipoproteins are the source of LDL cholesterol. The majority of these particles are cholesterol, which they carry to your body's cells. LDLs are often referred to as the "bad" cholesterol. Why? LDLs mean quite a bit to your body. However, when there are too many of them in your blood, they become harmful. They can build up on the walls of your arteries when they combine with other substances. Plaque is formed by these fatty deposits and grows over time. Atherosclerosis refers to the formation of plaque, and it increases your risk of heart disease, stroke, and other conditions.

You want to keep your LDL cholesterol level low. If you have a history of atherosclerosis, you should keep your LDL cholesterol below 70 mg/dL. This is the goal for the majority of adults

What is HDL cholesterol?

High-density lipoproteins are referred to as HDL cholesterol. Protein makes up the majority of these lipoproteins. HDL is the "good" cholesterol because it transports extra cholesterol to your liver from your bloodstream. Your liver then, at that point, separates the cholesterol and disposes of it. Reverse cholesterol transport is the name of this process.

Your HDL cholesterol is a number you need to keep high. An HDL of at least 60 is ideal for all adults and may lower your risk of heart disease. Assigned male at birth (AMAB) should aim for an HDL of at least 40 mg/dL. Assigned female at birth (AFAB) should aim for an HDL of at least 50 mg/dL.

What is VLDL cholesterol?

The term "very low-density lipoproteins" (VLDL cholesterol) is used. The protein content of VLDLs is low, and they contain cholesterol and triglycerides. As they're LDLs, they are "terrible" because they can add to plaque development in your corridors.

LDL cholesterol serves what purpose?

The term "bad cholesterol" is frequently applied to LDL cholesterol. Since LDL aids in the delivery of cholesterol to your cells, which is essential for your health, this is slightly oversimplified. However, there is a strong link between having too much LDL in your blood and a higher risk of heart disease.

This is because cholesterol plaque, or fatty deposits on your arteries, can result from high levels of LDL in your blood. Your blood vessels become more congested as a result, which is known as atherosclerosis. Your blood flow is affected, which can result in:

1. high cholesterol

2. chest discomfort (angina)

3. stroke

4. heart attack

5. ongoing kidney illness

It's essential to take note that this interaction happens over numerous years. There are numerous lifestyle changes you can make to help lower your LDL levels if you are aware that they are elevated. In a nutshell, you can do a lot to stop the process.

Many years of examination uphold the job LDL cholesterol can play in the advancement of coronary illness. However, only one of many elements adds to the improvement of coronary illness.

HDL cholesterol serves what purpose?

HDL cholesterol is frequently called "good cholesterol". This is because HDL aids in the transfer of LDL cholesterol from the arteries to the liver, where it can be eliminated from the body.

This process helps lower your risk of heart disease by stopping plaque from building up on the walls of your arteries. Your risk may rise if your HDL levels are too low.

VLDL cholesterol serves what purpose?

VLDL cholesterol is produced in your liver. VLDL transports fatty oils in your blood — where your body will either store the fatty substances or use them for energy. VLDL, like LDL cholesterol, is linked to plaque buildup in the arteries.

How to Check Your Cholesterol

A cholesterol blood test, also known as a lipid test, measures your LDL cholesterol, HDL cholesterol, total cholesterol, and triglyceride levels.

VLDL is difficult to directly measure. Your triglyceride levels are typically used by a laboratory to estimate your VLDL levels, which are typically approximately one-fifth of your triglyceride level.

By understanding which sorts of cholesterol are out of reach, you can zero in on way-of-life factors that can further develop each type explicitly.

How to Reduce LDL cholesterol in your diet

1. Eat food sources high in solvent fiber

Food sources like oats, kidney beans, Brussels fledglings, and apples contain solvent fiber. LDL cholesterol is "mopped up" by this type of fiber, which lowers levels.

2. Follow a Mediterranean diet.

This refers to the traditional diet of Mediterranean countries. While this kind of diet shifts by country, it's commonly high in natural products, vegetables, vegetables (like chickpeas), beans, nuts, entire grains, and fish. In addition, it has a lot of unsaturated fats, like olive oil. and typically contains little alcohol, dairy, or meat.

3. Engage in regular endurance training.

Exercise assists in moving LDL cholesterol to your liver, where it is eliminated. Public rules suggested 150 minutes of moderate-force or 75 minutes of extreme focus practice for seven days.

How to Lower VLDL Cholesterol.

Because triglyceride levels have a significant impact on VLDL cholesterol levels, lowering these will help lower VLDL cholesterol levels.

1. **Be mindful of what you eat**.

When you eat more calories than you need, your body makes triglycerides. Mindful eating can help prevent this. Mindful eating involves listening to your body's signals that you're hungry, eating slowly and thoroughly, considering how it makes you feel, and stopping when you feel full.

2. Quit Smoking and Alcohol

A recent study has found that smoking cigarettes lowers good cholesterol (HDL) levels in the blood and increases the likelihood of developing high blood pressure or diabetes. These conditions can lead to heart attack and stroke. However, smokers can lower their LDL cholesterol and raise their HDL cholesterol by giving up smoking.

Additionally, quitting smoking can help to protect arteries from damage. Nonsmokers should also avoid passive smoking to protect their health. Limit your alcohol intake, or don't drink at all. Study shows that alcohol can increase triglyceride and VLDL-C levels.

3. Consume sufficient omega-3 fats

Omega-3 fats may reduce triglyceride levels, blood pressure, and the risk of clotting. Slick fish, similar to salmon, is one of the most outstanding wellsprings of omega-3s. Omega-3 can be found in some plant foods like chia seeds and walnuts. However, this kind of omega-3 is harder for your body to use, so taking EPA/DHA supplements can help.

How to Make Your HDL Cholesterol Go Up

1. Regular high-intensity exercise has been linked to higher HDL cholesterol levels. You must engage in high-intensity exercise to achieve this beneficial effect; lower-intensity activities like walking do not appear to have the same effect.

2.   Try not to smoke

Smoking cigarettes is connected with lower HDL cholesterol levels, as well as influencing how well it can work. HDL levels can quickly rise after quitting smoking.

Chapter two

SYMPTOMS AND CAUSES OF HIGH CHOLESTEROL

Due to its close connection to cardiovascular diseases, high cholesterol has emerged as a significant cause for concern in severalty. Although cholesterol is necessary for several bodily functions, such as the formation of cell membranes and the production of hormones, elevated levels can pose serious health risks. We will examine the main factors that contribute to high cholesterol in this chapter, highlighting both lifestyle choices that can be changed and genetic predispositions.

People can take proactive measures to control their cholesterol levels and protect their cardiovascular health by comprehending these causes. The most common causes of high cholesterol are as follows:

1. Dietary Decisions:

One of the main sources of high cholesterol is an undesirable eating routine, especially one that is high in soaked and trans fats. These bad fats are abundant in commercially baked goods, red meat, full-fat dairy products, deep-fried snacks, and baked goods. These fats raise levels of low-density lipoprotein (LDL) cholesterol, also known as "bad" cholesterol, when consumed in large quantities. LDL cholesterol can build up in the arteries and form plaques that make it harder for blood to flow and make you more likely to get heart disease.

2. Lifestyle of Seclusion:

High cholesterol is significantly caused by a lack of physical activity. Customary activity has been displayed to build levels of high-Density lipoprotein (HDL) cholesterol, frequently alluded to as "good" cholesterol. HDL cholesterol aids in the removal of LDL cholesterol from the blood, lowering the likelihood of plaque formation. Conversely, a sedentary lifestyle results in lower HDL cholesterol levels, making it more difficult for the body to effectively regulate LDL cholesterol.

3. Obesity and weight gain:

High cholesterol levels are closely linked to obesity and excess weight. Cholesterol metabolism can be significantly affected by excess body fat, especially in the abdominal region. HDL cholesterol levels are lower and LDL cholesterol and triglyceride levels are frequently elevated in overweight or obese individuals. The unfavorable lipid profile created by these imbalances raises the risk of cardiovascular disease and atherosclerosis.

4. Family history of high cholesterol levels:

High cholesterol levels may be primarily inherited in some instances. Familial hypercholesterolemia (FH) is an acquired condition described by elevated degrees of LDL cholesterol from birth. Individuals with FH have a damaged or missing LDL receptor, prompting debilitated leeway of LDL cholesterol from the circulation system. As a result, people with FH have significantly elevated levels of LDL cholesterol, necessitating frequent medical intervention to effectively manage their condition.

5. Gender and age:

As people age, their cholesterol levels will generally rise. Because the lipid profile is negatively impacted by the decline in estrogen levels after menopause, this increase is more pronounced in women. Higher levels of LDL cholesterol and lower levels of HDL cholesterol can be caused by aging and the female gender, requiring increased management and awareness levels.

High cholesterol is caused by several different factors, including genetics and lifestyle choices that can be changed. An eating routine wealthy in unfortunate fats, stationary propensities, overabundance weight, and hereditary inclinations can all add to high cholesterol levels. However, individuals can effectively manage their cholesterol levels and lower their risk of cardiovascular diseases by adopting a heart-healthy lifestyle, which includes eating a well-balanced diet, engaging in regular physical activity, managing their weight, and seeking medical attention when necessary. Focusing on cholesterol on the board is a proactive move toward accomplishing ideal well-being and prosperity

Diseases and possible symptoms caused by high cholesterol are closely associated with numerous other health issues. This indicates that it may initially result in some serious issues, such as coronary artery disease. However, it can also occur as a result of other illnesses, particularly those that cause inflammation in the body (such as lupus). High cholesterol is frequently associated with high blood pressure as well.

What is high cholesterol?

Once more, high cholesterol is caused by having too many lipids (fats) in your blood. It is also known as hypercholesterolemia or hyperlipidemia. Your body needs a perfectly measured proportion of lipids to work. Your body can't use all of the lipids you have if you have too many. The additional lipids begin to accumulate in your arteries. They form plaque, which is a fatty deposit when they combine with other substances in your blood.

Although this plaque may not cause any issues for years, it silently grows larger and larger within your arteries over time. High cholesterol can be dangerous if left untreated. Without your knowledge, the extra lipids in your blood contribute to the plaque's expansion. A blood test is the only way to determine if you have high cholesterol.

You can find out how many lipids are circulating in your blood by having a blood test called a lipid panel. Your age, gender, and history of heart disease all play a role in determining what constitutes high cholesterol.

Lipids can be divided into good cholesterol and bad cholesterol. The terms "good cholesterol" and "bad cholesterol" are the most common.

High-density lipoprotein (HDL) is the name of the good cholesterol. Consider the "H" to mean "helpful." Cholesterol travels to your liver through your HDLs. Your liver keeps your cholesterol levels adjusted. It eliminates the remaining cholesterol and produces enough cholesterol to meet your body's needs. HDLs are essential for transporting cholesterol to the liver. You will have an excessive amount of cholesterol in your blood if your HDL levels are too low.

Awful cholesterol is called low-Density lipoprotein (LDL). This is the offender that makes plaque structure in your courses. Over time, heart disease can result from having too many LDLs

When to get checked for high cholesterol.

High cholesterol can begin in childhood or adolescence. Because of this, the current guidelines recommend starting screenings when children are young.

• Young people and teens:

Have your cholesterol looked at like clockwork beginning at age nine. A kid whose guardians have high cholesterol or a past filled with heart issues might start even sooner.

• Assigned male at birth (AMAB): Have your cholesterol looked at like clockwork until age 45. Get checked every one to two years from 45 to 65. Get checked every year after age 65.

• Assigned female at birth (AFAB): Until you are 55, get checked every five years. From age 55 to 65, get checked at least each one to two years. Get checked every year after age 65.

These are general recommendations. Your medical services supplier will examine what's best for you. For instance, a person in their 20s who has high cholesterol levels may require annual tests for some time. In addition, people who have other risk factors for heart disease may require more frequent tests.

Reasons for high cholesterol

Way of life variables and hereditary qualities both assume a part in causing high cholesterol. Some aspects of life include:

• Using tobacco and smoking:

Smoking brings down your "good cholesterol" (HDL) and raises your "bad cholesterol" (LDL).

• Feeling a lot of pressure:

Your body produces cholesterol as a result of hormonal changes brought about by stress.

• Consuming liquor:

Consuming an excessive amount of alcohol can raise total cholesterol.

• Not moving around enough:

Actual work like vigorous activity further develops your cholesterol numbers. Your body won't produce enough "good cholesterol" if you work at a desk or spend a lot of time sitting down in your spare time.

• Diet:

A few food varieties might raise or lower your cholesterol. At times medical care suppliers will suggest dietary changes or an encounter with a nutritionist to examine your eating regimen.

Side effects of high cholesterol

High cholesterol causes no side effects for the vast majority. You could be a long-distance runner and have high cholesterol. You won't begin to feel any side effects until the high cholesterol leads to different issues in your body.

Peripheral artery disease, high blood pressure, and stroke are all linked to high cholesterol. High cholesterol is also normal among individuals with diabetes.

How does my body respond to high cholesterol?

High cholesterol causes plaque to build up in your blood vessels over time. This plaque development is called atherosclerosis. Individuals with atherosclerosis face a higher gamble of various ailments. That is because your veins accomplish significant work all through your body. As a result, any issue with one of your blood vessels has a ripple effect.

You can consider your veins an intricate organization of lines that keep blood moving through your body. The gunk that clogs your home's pipes and slows down your shower drain is analogous to plaque. Plaque restricts blood flow by adhering to the inner walls of your blood vessels.

Plaque builds up inside your blood vessels when you have high cholesterol. The plaque grows larger the longer you go without treatment. Your blood vessels become narrowed or blocked as the plaque grows in size. Your blood vessels may continue to function for some time, analogous to a drain that is partially clogged. However, they won't work as well as they should. Depending on the clogged blood vessels, high cholesterol increases your risk of other medical conditions.

Coronary artery disease (CAD)

Coronary artery disease (CAD) is additionally called coronary illness or ischemic coronary illness. The majority of people mean this when they refer to heart disease. CAD is the leading cause of death and the most common type of heart disease in NIgeria and other parts of Africa and in the United States. CAD happens when atherosclerosis influences your coronary corridors. Your heart receives blood from these blood vessels. Your heart becomes weaker and stops working as it should when it doesn't get enough blood. Carotid artery disease can prompt a coronary episode or cardiovascular breakdown.

What many individuals don't know is that CAD can influence more youthful individuals. People under the age of 65 account for about one in five CAD deaths.

As a result, getting your cholesterol checked at a young age is critical. Plaque can silently accumulate in your coronary arteries over time. Until they experience chest pain (angina) or another sign of a heart attack, many people don't realize it's happening.

Carotid artery disease occurs when your carotid arteries are impacted by atherosclerosis. The carotid arteries in your neck carry blood to your large, frontal brain. Your brain doesn't get enough oxygen-rich blood when plaque narrows these arteries. A stroke or a transient ischemic attack (TIA, also known as a "mini-stroke") can result from carotid artery disease.

Peripheral artery disease (PAD)

Peripheral artery disease (PAD) occurs when atherosclerosis affects the arteries in your arms or legs. Because they are away from your heart and the center of your body, the arteries in your legs and arms are considered to be "peripheral." Although PAD can occur in your arms as well, it is more prevalent in your legs.

The cushion is perilous because it frequently causes no side effects. You could at long last begin to feel side effects when a fringe corridor is no less than 60% hindered. Intermittent claudication is a significant symptom. This is a leg cramp that fires up while you're moving around however at that point stops when you rest. It's a sign that plaque in your artery is making it harder for blood to flow.

PAD can cause significant issues not only in your legs and feet but also in other parts of your body. This is because your cardiovascular system connects all of your blood vessels. Therefore, plaque buildup in one area slows down your entire "pipe" network.

Although they are not the same thing, PAD and coronary artery disease (CAD) are related. It is likely that people with one condition also have the other. Numerous risk factors are the same for PAD and CAD.

High cholesterol and high blood pressure (hypertension) are linked conditions. Your arteries become hard and narrow as a result of cholesterol plaque and calcium. As a result, getting blood through them takes a lot more effort from your heart. Your blood pressure rises too high as a result.

Heart disease is primarily brought on by two factors: high cholesterol and high blood pressure. About one in three adults in Nigeria and in the United States have high cholesterol and high blood pressure. For the greater part of the grown-ups in each gathering, treatment isn't helping enough, or probably they're not utilizing any treatment.

Your doctor's medications can be very helpful, but making changes to your lifestyle can make them work better. Changing one's lifestyle is important for controlling both high blood pressure and cholesterol. Among the changes are:

• Eat less immersed fat and trans-fat:

Inexpensive food can contain high measures of both. However, depending on how they are prepared, even meals served in formal restaurants may contain a lot of saturated fat.

• Eat less seared food sources and handled food varieties: These incorporate prepackaged pastries and bites.

• Cut back on salt (sodium):

There are foods with hidden salt. Perusing marks in the store is significant. Nutritional information for menu items may be available for sharing in some restaurants.

• Stop using tobacco products and smoking: Smoking is a major risk factor for heart disease and problems with the blood vessels.

Your cholesterol levels are affected by what medical conditions?

Clinical issues and cholesterol have a two-way relationship. Atherosclerosis and other medical issues can result from high cholesterol. However, you may also be more likely to develop high cholesterol if you have certain medical conditions. Your cholesterol levels may be affected by the following conditions.

Ongoing kidney infection (CKD)

Individuals with an ongoing kidney infection (CKD) face a higher gamble of creating coronary vein illness. This is because CKD causes plaque to build up in their arteries more quickly. Heart disease is more likely to kill people with early-stage CKD than kidney disease.

Triglycerides, a type of fat, are more common in people with chronic kidney disease. Additionally, it makes your very low-density lipoprotein (VLDL) cholesterol levels rise. Triglyceride-carrying particles are known as VLDLs. In the meantime, CKD brings down your "good cholesterol" (HDL) levels and keeps your HDLs from functioning as they ought to. CKD additionally changes the construction of your "bad cholesterol" (LDL) particles so they truly hurt more.

HIV

The risk of having a heart attack or stroke is nearly twice as high in HIV-positive individuals as it is in non-HIV-positive ones. Analysts used to think this higher gamble came from HIV meds (antiretroviral treatment). They thought that taking those drugs made a person's cholesterol go up. However, more recent studies indicate that a person's immune system is actually to blame.

Your immune system may still be activated despite HIV treatment. Your body experiences chronic inflammation as a result of this. Atherosclerosis and plaque buildup are sparked by this inflammation.

The positive news is that HIV-positive individuals are living longer. However, this indicates that additional research is required to investigate their effects on chronic diseases like heart disease.

Cholesterol levels can be affected by thyroid disease. This is because your body processes lipids (fats) differently depending on the thyroid hormone. The effect is determined by your type of thyroid disease.

• Hyperthyroidism: Your body makes too much thyroid hormone as a result of this condition. Cholesterol levels (total, LDL, and HDL) can rise when you take medication to treat this condition. Discuss cholesterol management with your healthcare provider if you are receiving treatment for hyperthyroidism.

• Hypothyroidism: This condition makes your body make too minimal thyroid chemicals. It likewise makes you have more elevated cholesterol levels. Your cholesterol levels go down as a result of thyroid disease treatment in this instance. You might, in any case, have to take statins to get your cholesterol in the best reach. Your provider will talk about what's best for your particular situation.

Heart disease and thyroid disease are still being studied by researchers. A few examinations demonstrate the way that thyroid sickness can cause heart issues inconsequential to cholesterol or plaque development. Hyperthyroidism and hypothyroidism, for instance, may increase a person's risk of heart failure.

Lupus

Individuals with lupus generally have more significant levels of "terrible cholesterol" (LDL, VLDL) and fatty substances. Additionally, their "good cholesterol" (HDL) levels are lower. Individuals who have dynamic lupus face a more serious gamble of elevated cholesterol contrasted with the people who have very much made-due (calm) lupus.

Lupus raises your gamble of creating coronary corridor illness. This is because lupus causes chronic inflammation in the body. Your arteries' plaque buildup accelerates as a result of this inflammation.

Polycystic ovary syndrome (PCOS) People who have PCOS are more likely to develop heart disease. This chance goes up more as they age. PCOS raises the gamble of numerous coronary illness risk factors, including diabetes and hypertension. Low levels of "good cholesterol" (HDL) and high levels of "bad cholesterol" (LDL) are more common in PCOS sufferers.

Diabetes mellitus (both Type 1 and Type 2 diabetes) increases your risk of coronary and peripheral artery disease by twofold. Diabetes is connected with lower levels of HDLs and more elevated levels of fatty oils and LDLs.

Dyslipidemia related to diabetes affects roughly seven out of every ten people with Type 2 diabetes. This implies they have high fatty substance levels, high "little thick" LDL levels, and low HDL levels. " Little thick" LDL is a particular kind of cholesterol protein that can undoubtedly enter your corridor wall and cause harm. Plaque can form if there are too many small, dense LDLs in your blood. The relationship between diabetes and heart disease is still being investigated by researchers.

Ways to lower your cholesterol?

Discuss the most effective means of lowering your cholesterol with your healthcare provider. Some people only require minor lifestyle adjustments, such as consuming less saturated fat. Others require medication and lifestyle changes. A more complex approach may be required for individuals with cholesterol-lowering medical conditions. Consult with your supplier about your clinical history, family ancestry, and way of life factors. You will devise a strategy to lower your cholesterol levels together.

Recollect that even the best plans get some margin to work. And we all experience setbacks. It is acceptable to struggle and to inform your healthcare provider when a plan is not performing as expected. Sometimes, even making the most drastic changes to your lifestyle doesn't lower your cholesterol levels enough. This is because your liver is the source of most of your body's cholesterol.

As a result, a lot of other things happen that you can't control and have nothing to do with what's on your dinner plate.

Approach things slowly and carefully, and recollect that having elevated cholesterol is certainly not an individual disappointment. It is the result of numerous subtle changes taking place within your body. Be aware that medications and other medical interventions are available to fill in the gaps, so take control of what you can.

Cholesterol levels are silent and sneaky. You may not know you have too many lipids in your blood for a long time. A straightforward blood test is the best way to find out. All ages are affected by high cholesterol, even those who exercise regularly and feel healthy. A person's risk of heart disease and high cholesterol is increased by certain medical conditions. Learn about your numbers and discuss what they mean for you with your service provider.

Chapter three

The most effective method to oversee cholesterol level

Cholesterol is a waxy, fat-like substance tracked down in each cell of our body. Although cholesterol is needed by the body for several important functions, having too much of it can cause serious health issues like heart disease and stroke. Maintaining good overall health and lowering the risk of these conditions requires controlling cholesterol levels. In this chapter, we'll look at effective strategies and changes to your lifestyle that can help you control your cholesterol and keep your heart healthy.

❖ **Learn about cholesterol:**

Understanding the various types of cholesterol and their effects on health is essential for effective cholesterol management. Cholesterol can be broken down into two categories: cholesterol with a low density (LDL), also known as "bad" cholesterol, and cholesterol with a high density (HDL), also known as "good" cholesterol. HDL cholesterol helps remove LDL cholesterol from the bloodstream, whereas LDL cholesterol can build up in your arteries and raise your risk of heart disease.

❖ **Get checked for cholesterol:**

The first step in effectively managing cholesterol is knowing your levels. To find out your total cholesterol, LDL cholesterol, HDL cholesterol, and triglyceride levels, schedule a cholesterol screening with your doctor. This gauge estimation will assist you with laying out fitting objectives and keep tabs on your development after some time.

❖ **Follow a heart-friendly diet:**

Cholesterol levels can be controlled in large part through diet. Include the following healthy eating habits in your routine:

a. Cut back on trans and saturated fats:

 Limit your admission of soaked fats tracked down in red meat, full-fat dairy items, and tropical oils. Trans fats are typically found in fried and processed foods. Supplant these undesirable fats with better choices, for example, unsaturated fats tracked down in olive oil, avocados, and nuts.

b. Increase Consumption of Soluble Fiber:

Oats, barley, fruits, and vegetables, all of which are high in soluble fiber, can assist in lowering LDL cholesterol levels.

c. Eat fish high in omega-3 fatty acids:

Omega-3 unsaturated fats found in greasy fish like salmon, mackerel, and sardines have been displayed to lessen LDL cholesterol levels. If you hate fish, consider fish oil supplements.

d.   Eat Plant Sterols and Stanols:

LDL cholesterol can be reduced by these naturally occurring compounds in plants. Margarine and other foods enriched with plant sterols or stanols can be beneficial.

e. Reduce cholesterol in your diet:

Albeit dietary cholesterol affects blood cholesterol more than soaked and trans fats, consuming it in moderation is as yet prudent. Limit your admission to cholesterol-rich food varieties like organ meats and egg yolks.

❖ Keep a Solid Weight:

High cholesterol levels are caused by excess body weight. By accomplishing and keeping a solid weight, you can further develop your cholesterol profile. To support cardiovascular health and shed excess pounds, combine a well-balanced diet with regular exercise. In order to keep your wait on check, you can try out the following:

a.   Calorie Control:

Consume enough calories for your age, gender, and level of activity. Make progress toward a calorie balance that permits slow, supportable weight reduction if necessary.

b. Control of portions:

To avoid overeating, pay attention to portion sizes. Visual portion control is made easier by serving food on smaller plates, bowls, and utensils.

c. Consistent Activity:

Participate in normal oxygen-consuming activities, like lively strolling, cycling, or swimming, for no less than 150 minutes a week. Strength training exercises can help you build muscle, which in turn helps you burn calories more effectively.

❖ Engage in Activity:

Not only does physical activity help people lose weight, but it also directly lowers cholesterol levels. Customary activity can expand HDL cholesterol, diminish LDL cholesterol, and work on generally speaking cardiovascular well-being.

a. Aerobic Activities:

To increase your heart rate and improve your cardiovascular fitness, participate in aerobic activities like jogging, dancing, or sports.

b.   Strength Preparing:

Strengthening your muscles can be accomplished through resistance training with weights or resistance bands. Muscles that are strong support a healthy weight and help burn more calories.

c.   Lifestyle Changes:

Simplify changes to increment actual work over the day, like using the staircase rather than the lift, strolling or cycling for brief excursions, or taking part in dynamic leisure activities like cultivating or moving.

❖ Give up smoking:

Smoking causes damage to blood vessels, lowers HDL cholesterol levels, and raises the risk of cardiovascular disease. There are numerous health benefits to quitting smoking, including lower cholesterol levels and improved cardiovascular health as a whole. Look for help from medical care experts, support gatherings, or smoking discontinuance projects to stop smoking effectively.

❖ Reduce your alcohol intake:

While moderate alcohol consumption may have some benefits for the cardiovascular system, excessive alcohol consumption can raise blood pressure and triglyceride levels. Limit liquor utilization to direct levels

Reduce Stress:

Cholesterol levels and heart health as a whole can be affected by chronic stress. Engaging in hobbies, spending time with loved ones, getting enough sleep, and practicing relaxation techniques like deep breathing, meditation, and yoga are all healthy ways to manage stress.

❖ **Supplements and medications:**

Modifications to one's lifestyle may not always be enough to control cholesterol levels. To help you control your cholesterol, your doctor may prescribe cholesterol-lowering medications like statins. Follow your physician's instructions and take your medications as directed. Additionally, some supplements, such as red yeast rice, garlic extract, and plant sterols, may modestly lower cholesterol; however, you should always consult your doctor before beginning any supplements.

Maintaining good cardiovascular health necessitates managing cholesterol levels. You can effectively manage your cholesterol levels and lower your risk of heart disease by following a heart-healthy diet, maintaining a healthy weight, engaging in regular physical activity, and adopting healthy lifestyle habits. Keep in mind that the best way to control your cholesterol levels is to speak with your doctor. Make your heart health a priority and take action to live a healthier life.

Chapter four

How to lower cholesterol naturally

An individual's eating routine assumes a critical part in their cholesterol levels - a few food varieties can increase cholesterol, while others lower it. Several health problems can be avoided by maintaining healthy cholesterol levels. Cholesterol is a waxy substance that moves through the circulatory system as a piece of two lipoproteins: high-density lipoprotein and low-density lipoprotein

Because it contributes to the formation of fatty deposits in the blood vessels, LDL cholesterol is sometimes referred to as "bad" cholesterol. These stores can obstruct Believed Source bloodstream and cause coronary failures or strokes.

HDL, or "good" cholesterol, aids in the liver's removal of cholesterol from the body. HDL cholesterol can lower the likelihood of heart disease and stroke.

This part records food varieties that an individual can integrate into their eating regimen to further develop their cholesterol levels normally.

1. Eggplant

Eggplant is high in dietary fiber: 3 grams (g) of fiber are contained in a 100-gram serving. The American Heart Association (AHA) notes that fiber aids in lowering cholesterol levels in the blood. Additionally, it lowers the likelihood of:

- coronary illness
- stroke
- stoutness
- type 2 diabetes

2. Okra

People cultivate okra, also known as lady's fingers, a warm-season vegetable worldwide. Scientists have found that a gel in okra called adhesive can assist with bringing cholesterol by restricting it during processing. This makes it easier for cholesterol to leave the body through feces.

3.   Apples:

A   study showed that eating two apples a day reduced LDL cholesterol levels in 40 people with mildly elevated cholesterol. It likewise brought down degrees of fatty substances, a sort of fat in the blood.

Depending on its size, an apple may contain 3–7 g of dietary fiber. Additionally, apples contain polyphenols, which may have a beneficial effect on cholesterol levels.

4. Avocado

Avocados are wealthy in heart-solid supplements. According to a 2015 study, consuming one avocado per day as part of a diet low in cholesterol and low in fat can reduce the risk of cardiovascular disease, particularly LDL cholesterol, but not HDL cholesterol.

Monounsaturated fats, which can lower LDL cholesterol levels and lower the risk of heart disease and stroke, can be found in 150 grams (or one cup) of avocado.

5. Fish

Omega-3 fats, for example, eicosatetraenoic corrosive (EPA), are fundamental polyunsaturated fats tracked down in fish like salmon, mackerel, and sardines, with proven and factual calming and heart medical advantages.

EPA can assist with shielding the veins and heart from illness by bringing down degrees of fatty oils, a fat that enters the circulation system after dinner. It may reduce the risk of cardiovascular disease and prevent atherosclerosis in several ways, including this one.

Other heart medical advantages incorporate keeping cholesterol gems from framing in the supply routes, diminishing irritation, and further developing the way that HDL cholesterol works.

6. oats

oats significantly reduced blood cholesterol levels. 70 grams of oats in the form of porridge were consumed daily by some people with mildly elevated cholesterol levels. According to research, this provided them with 3 g of soluble fiber per day, which is the amount required to lower cholesterol.

As part of a heart-healthy diet, Other Source confirms that oats' soluble fiber can lower LDL cholesterol levels and reduce cardiovascular risk.

Oats can be added to a person's diet by eating porridge or cereal made with oats for breakfast.

7. Barley

Barley is a nutritious grain that is high in fiber and contains a lot of vitamins and minerals. According to the findings of a 2018 study, beta-glucan, a type of soluble dietary fiber found in oats and barley may assist in lowering LDL cholesterol.

A 2020 study provided additional insight into this process. By limiting the amount of cholesterol the body absorbs during digestion and trapping bile acids, the team discovered that beta-glucan reduces LDL cholesterol.

The body uses cholesterol to make bile acids to replace those that are stuck, which lowers cholesterol levels overall.

Barley's beta-glucan also improves blood glucose control and the microbiome in the gut, which is beneficial to heart health.

8. Nuts

Nuts are a good source of unsaturated fats, which can help lower LDL cholesterol, especially when they are consumed in place of saturated fats. Additionally, nuts are high in fiber, which aids in the elimination of cholesterol and prevents the body from absorbing it. All nuts are reasonable for a heart-solid, cholesterol-bringing-down diet, including:

Cashews, Brazil nuts, almonds, walnuts, pistachios, pecans, hazelnuts, and Soy. If you want to lower your cholesterol, you can eat soy products like tofu, soy milk, and soy yogurt. According to a 2019 review of 46 studies on how soy affects LDL cholesterol, consuming 25 g of soy protein per day for six weeks reduced LDL cholesterol by a clinically significant 4.76 milligrams per deciliter. Overall, the researchers concluded that adults' LDL cholesterol can be reduced by 3–4% with soy protein, establishing its place in a diet that is good for the heart and lowers cholesterol.

9. Dark chocolate Cocoa, which can be found in dark chocolate, contains flavonoids, which are a group of compounds that can be found in a wide variety of vegetables and fruits. There are numerous ways that their antioxidant and anti-inflammatory properties can benefit health.

For a month, some people consumed cocoa-flavanol-containing beverages twice daily. Their HDL cholesterol levels had increased and their LDL cholesterol levels had decreased by the trial's conclusion. However, dark chocolate products should be consumed in moderation due to their high sugar and saturated fat content.

10. Lentils

Lentils are wealthy in fiber, containing 3.3g per 100-g segment. Fiber can keep the body from retaining cholesterol in the circulation system. The positive effects of eating lentils on cholesterol levels were demonstrated by a study that included 39 overweight or obese people with type 2 diabetes. HDL levels increased, while LDL and triglyceride levels decreased after eight weeks of eating 60 grams of lentil sprouts daily.

11. Garlic

Garlic can be used in a variety of dishes and has numerous health benefits. For instance, scientists have found that garlic can assist with managing serum cholesterol levels. What's more, another Source confirmed that garlic can likewise assist with lessening circulatory strain. However, these studies used supplements of garlic, and it would be difficult to consume enough garlic to have a significant impact on cholesterol levels.

12. Green tea

Some teas, like green tea, contain antioxidants known as catechins that can be very good for your health. A trusted Source found that green tea utilization fundamentally further developed cholesterol levels, lessening both aggregate and LDL cholesterol levels without bringing down HDL cholesterol levels. To confirm their findings, the researchers call for additional research.

14. Extra virgin olive oil

The heart-healthy Mediterranean diet frequently includes extra virgin olive oil. One of its many purposes is as a cooking oil. Low-density lipoprotein (LDL) levels may be reduced by replacing butter's saturated fat with extra virgin olive oil's monounsaturated fat.

Additionally, the antioxidant and anti-inflammatory properties of extra virgin olive oil can be extremely beneficial to cardiovascular and overall health.

14. Kale

Kale is a brilliant wellspring of fiber and numerous different supplements. Fiber can be found in one cup of boiled kale. A 2016 review demonstrated a link between lower blood pressure and lower levels of fat in the blood. Remembering more fiber for the eating routine can assist with bringing down degrees of absolute cholesterol and LDL cholesterol. Antioxidants, which are beneficial to the heart and aid in reducing inflammation, can also be found in kale.

Cholesterol-bringing down diet plan

The following are a few thoughts for dinners that might assist with further developing cholesterol levels:

Breakfast

- apple and peanut butter on entire-grain toast

- cinnamon oats and low-fat plain Greek yogurt

- oats with blueberries and almonds

Lunch

- vegetables and hummus in entire-grain pita

- Mediterranean vegetable stew with grain

• Kale salad finished off with edamame and avocado

Dinner

- poached salmon with asparagus and brown rice

- lentil stew with salsa Verde

- entire wheat pasta with chicken and Brussels sprouts thrown in olive oil

Snacks

Attempt the accompanying snacks with some restraint as a component of a cholesterol-bringing-down diet:

Whole grain pretzels or crackers, roasted chickpeas or edamame, rye crisps with tuna, low-fat or fat-free yogurt, a handful of pistachios or another nut, apple slices with almond butter, and a granola bar made from oats, nuts, and dried fruit are all good options.

Chapter five

Drinks that help lower or control cholesterol levels

Compounds found in a wide variety of beverages have the potential to reduce or manage cholesterol levels. Oat drinks, soy drinks, plant milk smoothies, and green tea are all examples. The body uses cholesterol, a waxy substance, to make hormones and cells. There are two distinct types of cholesterol: high-density lipoprotein (HDL) and low-density lipoprotein (LDL).

At the point when cholesterol levels are unhealthful, it expands the gamble of serious ailments, for example, stroke or coronary episodes. We'll talk about drinks to avoid and drinks that might help you control your cholesterol levels in this chapter. Additionally, this chapter will provide a list of alternative strategies that may be beneficial to individuals aiming for healthier cholesterol levels.

Best drinks to lower cholesterol. Numerous drinks can lower or control cholesterol. These are some

Green tea

Green tea contains catechins and other cancer prevention agents that help lower "terrible" LDL and absolute cholesterol levels. In 2015, researchers gave drinking water infused with catechins and epigallocatechin gallate—an additional helpful antioxidant found in green tea—to rats.

The two groups of rats on high-cholesterol diets had cholesterol and "bad" LDL levels that had decreased by approximately 14.4% and

30.4% after 56 days, respectively. However, to investigate this further, additional human studies are required.

Although black tea is less beneficial than its green counterpart, it can still have a beneficial effect on cholesterol. This is primarily because the body absorbs liquid differently when there are different amounts of catechins in the teas. Caffeine may also assist in raising HDL levels.

Soy milk

Soy contains little saturated fat. Soy milk or creamers, in place of cream or high-fat milk products, may aid in cholesterol management. To lower the risk of heart disease, the Food and Drug Administration (FDA) suggests including soy protein in a diet low in cholesterol and saturated fat.

Also, it is desirable to consume soy in its entire and negligibly handled structure with next to zero added sugars, salts, and fats. A few specialists suggest polishing off 2-3 servings of soy-based food sources or beverages day to day, with one serving to address 250 milliliters (ml) of soy milk.

Oat drinks

Oats contain beta-glucans, which make a gel-like substance in the stomach and communicate with bile salts, which hinder cholesterol retention and assist with diminishing cholesterol levels. An investigation discovered that oat drinks, for example, oat milk, may offer a more reliable decrease in cholesterol than semi-strong or strong oat items. Oat milk can provide 1 gram of beta-glucans in 250 milliliters.

Make a point to check out drink marks to guarantee they contain beta-glucans, which might show up as a component of the fiber data, and the amount they incorporate per serving.

Tomato juice

Tomatoes are wealthy in a compound called lycopene, which might further develop lipid levels and lessen "terrible" LDL cholesterol. Additionally, research indicates that juicing tomatoes raises their lycopene content. Niacin and fiber that lowers cholesterol are also abundant in tomato juice. 25 women who consumed 280 milliliters of tomato juice daily for two months experienced a decrease in blood cholesterol levels, according to a 2015 study.

Smoothies made with berries:

A lot of berries are full of antioxidants and fiber, both of which may lower cholesterol levels. Anthocyanins, a potent antioxidant found in berries, have been shown to lower cholesterol. Additionally, berries are low in fat and calories. Blend two handfuls, or about 80 grams, of any berry to make a berry smoothie. Add half a cup of ice water and half a cup of low-fat milk or yogurt to the berries.

Berries that are particularly beneficial to health include:

• blackberries, blueberries, raspberries, and strawberries Drinks with sterols and stanols. Sterols and stanols are plant chemicals that block the absorption of some cholesterol. They are similar to cholesterol in shape and size. Vegetables and nuts, on the other hand, do not contain any sterols or stanols that can lower cholesterol. These chemicals are being added by companies to a variety of foods and drinks, such as yogurt drinks, fruit juices, fortified plant-based spreads, and milk.

The Food and Drug Administration (FDA) recommends that the majority of people aim to consume 3.4 g of stanols and 1.3 g of sterols per day. Try to consume these sterols and stanols with a meal if you can.

Drinks made of cocoa

Cocoa is the primary component of dark chocolate. Flavanols, which doctors refer to as antioxidants, may lower cholesterol levels. A drink containing 450 mg of cocoa flavanols was found to lower "bad" LDL cholesterol and increase "good" HDL cholesterol when taken twice daily for a month. Monounsaturated fatty acids, which can also help lower cholesterol, are abundant in cocoa. However, beverages with processed chocolate in them contain a lot of saturated fat. Limit chocolate with added sugars, salts, and fats for healthy alternatives.

Smoothies made with plant milk

Many varieties of plant-based milk contain components that have the potential to lower or control cholesterol levels. An individual can make a reasonable smoothie base utilizing soy milk or oat milk. Make a soy or oat smoothie by mixing 1 cup (250 ml) of soy or oat milk with cholesterol-bringing down natural products or vegetables, for example,

• 1 banana

• 1 handful of grapes or prunes

• 1 slice of mango or melon

• 2 small plums

• 1 cup of kale or Swiss chard

• 1/3 cup pumpkin puree

Not to Drink by People who want to lower their cholesterol levels or keep their health at a healthy level may want to avoid beverages that are high in saturated fats, such as:

Drinks or smoothies containing coconut or palm oils; pressed coconut drinks; ice-cream-based drinks; high-fat milk products; coffees or teas with cream, whipped cream, high-fat milk, or creamer added. Drinking more than 12 ounces of sugary drinks per day may also lower HDL levels and raise triglyceride levels, or levels of fat in the blood.

Beverages that are sweetened with sugar include:

• fruit juices; sports drinks; energy drinks; soda or pop; sweetened coffees or teas; hot chocolate; prepackaged smoothies; chocolate or sweetened milk products. Some studies have found that drinking moderate amounts of alcohol may be better for heart health than not drinking at all.

Moderate liquor utilization might assist with expanding "great" HDL cholesterol levels. Females should consume no more than one alcoholic beverage per day and men should consume no more than two. However, a person's age, sex, and the kind of alcohol they consume all play a significant role in determining how alcohol affects cholesterol levels. Additionally, excessive drinking raises cholesterol, and there are so many health risks associated with alcohol consumption that the risks likely outweigh the benefits.

Cooking Methods and Tips

Explicit cooking strategies can change the soaked fat substance in a feast. A few simple acclimations to make to cooking schedules include:

Cutting off all visible fat from meat and removing the skin from poultry before cooking

• Skimming off the top layer of congealed fat after the soup has been refrigerated

• Using wine instead of fat drippings to baste meat

• using a rack to drain off fat when broiling, roasting, or baking poultry or meats

• cutting off all visible fat from meat and removing the skin from poultry before cooking

• skimming off the top layer of congealed fat after the soup has been ref

Cholesterol is a substance that looks like fat and is made by the body in high quantities on its own. A good way to control cholesterol levels is to avoid foods high in trans and unsaturated fats. Red meat, skinless poultry, and full-fat dairy products are all cholesterol- and fat-rich foods.

Consuming a solid eating regimen wealthy in fiber, entire foods grown from the ground, and lean protein sources can assist an individual with keeping up with ideal cholesterol levels and advance general well-being.

Chapter six

Foods to Avoid and foods to Eat:

If you have high cholesterol, it is essential to limit your enthusiasm for certain foods while continuing to consume others regularly. Here is a gander at two sorts of food varieties to eat and three to stay away from for high cholesterol victims notwithstanding what we have examined before in this book.

Dairy Products

It's easy to make the mistake of thinking that eggs should be avoided if you're watching your cholesterol because they contain cholesterol. However, according to Healthline, eggs are full of nutrients and can increase HDLs, which are good for the heart and should be consumed in moderation. Despite their high B12 content, eggs are high in cholesterol. Essentially, full-fat cheddar and yogurt are still up in the air to be a sound dietary decision, regardless of whether you have high cholesterol, reports Healthline.

High Fiber Food

Dissolvable fiber has been displayed to assist with diminishing degrees of "terrible" LDL cholesterol, and that implies you ought to eat bunches of foods grown from the ground, including salad greens and different vegetables high in leptin. These high-soluble food varieties help to decrease aggravation.

When you go grocery shopping, make it a habit to buy a lot of fresh produce. If you're not very good at cooking, learn how to cook vegetables in healthy ways. Oatmeal and other cereals high in soluble fiber are excellent choices for breakfast, and if you have high cholesterol, you should eat beans and other legumes frequently, according to Healthline.

Shellfish

Loaded with protein, B nutrients, and iron, shellfish are nutritious and great to eat if you have high cholesterol, as per Healthline. They are a good source of taurine and antioxidants from carotenoids, both of which aid in lowering LDL cholesterol. Healthline adds that people with high cholesterol can still enjoy clams, shrimp, crab, and oysters as long as they are broiled, steamed, or cooked in oil that is good for the heart. Note that shellfish are viewed as food varieties high in purines and ought to stay away from assuming you're a gout victim, as per the Joint Pain

Establishment.

According to Reader's Digest, fried foods like fish sticks, French fries, and chicken fingers may taste delicious, but these high-cholesterol deep-fried foods are often loaded with trans fats and should be avoided if you have high cholesterol. Except for special occasions, you should drive right by your favorite fast-food restaurant. Healthline reports that consumption of fried foods is associated with an increased risk of heart disease and obesity.

Sugary Desserts:

Who doesn't like ice cream, cookies, and muffins? A reliable Source says that while sugary desserts can't be completely avoided, they should be limited if you have high cholesterol. According to Healthline, these foods not only make you gain weight, but they also frequently contain unhealthy fats and lack essential nutrients. All things being equal, eat a new natural product, yogurt that is low in sugar, or a square of dim chocolate as an after-supper treat.

DISCLAIMER!

All the information provided in this book is based on medical research. This book is to provide you with basic things you need to know about Cholesterol.

However, if you have any health challenge, please ensure to see your doctor for proper medical advice.